New and Emerging Areas in Medicine Series

Diversity, Equity, and Inclusion Competencies Across the Learning Continuum

Association of American Medical Colleges
Washington, D.C.

The AAMC (Association of American Medical Colleges) is a nonprofit association dedicated to improving the health of people everywhere through medical education, health care, medical research, and community collaborations. Its members comprise all 155 accredited U.S. and 16 accredited Canadian medical schools; approximately 400 teaching hospitals and health systems, including Department of Veterans Affairs medical centers; and more than 70 academic societies. Through these institutions and organizations, the AAMC leads and serves America's medical schools and teaching hospitals and the millions of individuals employed across academic medicine, including more than 191,000 full-time faculty members, 95,000 medical students, 149,000 resident physicians, and 60,000 graduate students and postdoctoral researchers in the biomedical sciences. In 2022, the Association of Academic Health Centers and the Association of Academic Health Centers International merged into the AAMC, broadening the AAMC's U.S. membership and expanding its reach to international academic health centers. Learn more at aamc.org.

Suggested citation: AAMC. *Diversity, Equity, and Inclusion Competencies Across the Learning Continuum.* AAMC New and Emerging Areas in Medicine Series. Washington, DC: AAMC; 2022.

ISBN: 978-1-57754-206-3

Contents

Preface

Health care is changing rapidly. New technologies, advances in care delivery, and scientific discoveries are happening at rates that make it challenging for teaching and learning practices across the continuum to keep up. Whether learners are at the beginning of their career or seasoned clinicians, new demands and advances in health care require them to acquire new competencies. The AAMC New and Emerging Areas in Medicine Series is a guide for everyone who develops curricula within the field of medicine and for people learning to practice or continuing their professional development.

"The AAMC New and Emerging Areas in Medicine Series is a guide for everyone who develops curricula within the field of medicine and for people learning to practice or continuing their professional development."

Each set of new and emerging competencies is developed by leaders from across the medical education and clinical practice communities, including hundreds of reviewers of iterative drafts who provided input through surveys and focus groups. These competencies add depth to selected emerging areas to help guide curricular and professional development, formative performance assessment, cross-continuum collaborations, and, ultimately, improvements in health care services and outcomes. They are not intended for high-stakes assessment or for purposes of accreditation. This series includes competencies in quality improvement and patient safety (QIPS), telehealth, and now, with this report, diversity, equity, and inclusion (DEI).

Acknowledgments

The AAMC acknowledges the dedication of the talented members of the Diversity, Equity, and Inclusion Advisory Committee, who helped develop and revise draft competencies, and the hundreds of students, residents, faculty, affiliates, patient advocates, and others who reviewed drafts throughout the iterative development process. We thank them for their dedication to advancing DEI through education and collaboration across the continuum.

DIVERSITY, EQUITY, AND INCLUSION ADVISORY COMMITTEE, 2019-2021

Kendall Campbell, MD
Senior Associate Dean for Academic Affairs
Brody School of Medicine at East Carolina University

Cliff Coleman, MD, MPH
Associate Professor of Family Medicine
Oregon Health & Science University
School of Medicine

Chiquita A. Collins, PhD
Chief Diversity Officer, Vice Dean for Inclusion and Diversity
University of Texas Health Science Center at San Antonio
Joe R. and Teresa Lozano Long School of Medicine

Austyn Holleman, MSW, MPH, LGSW
Manager of Senior Mental Health Project
Mary's Center, Washington, D.C.

Aletha Maybank, MD, MPH
Chief Health Equity Officer
American Medical Association

William McDade, MD, PhD
Chief Diversity and Inclusion Officer
Accreditation Council for Graduate Medical Education

David McIntosh, PhD, MA
Vice Dean for Justice, Equity, Diversity, and Inclusion
University of California, Los Angeles,
David Geffen School of Medicine

Michelle Morse, MD, MPH
Instructor in Medicine, Co-Founder,
Social Medicine Consortium
Harvard Medical School

Jann Murray-García, MD, MPH
Associate Clinical Professor,
Betty Irene Moore School of Nursing
UC Davis Health

Beth Nelson, MD
Associate Dean of Undergraduate Medical Education
University of Texas at Austen Dell Medical School

Ann-Gel Palermo, DrPH, MPH
Associate Dean for Diversity and Inclusion
in Biomedical Education
Icahn School of Medicine at Mount Sinai

Brenda Pereda, MD
Assistant Dean for Diversity, Equity and Inclusion
University of New Mexico School of Medicine

Jennifer E. Potter, MD
Advisory Dean and Director of the William B. Castle Society
Beth Israel Deaconess Medical Center

José E. Rodríguez, MD, FAAFP
Associate Vice President for Health Equity and Inclusion
University of Utah Health

Lawrence K. Rolle, MD, MBA
Combined Internal Medicine and Pediatrics Resident
University of Miami, Jackson, Memorial Hospital
Medical Student Representative
Keck School of Medicine of the University of Southern California

Richard deShazo, MD
Emeritus Professor of Medicine and Pediatrics
University of Alabama at Birmingham
Marnix E. Heersink School of Medicine

Jeffrey Uribe, MD
Emergency Medical Service Fellow
Newark Beth Israel

Donald Warne, MD, MPH
Associate Dean of Diversity, Equity and Inclusion
University of North Dakota School of Medicine
and Health Sciences

AAMC STAFF

David Acosta, MD
Chief Diversity and Inclusion Officer
Executive Co-Sponsor

Adrien Barrios
Program Specialist, Strategic Initiatives and Partnerships

Malika Fair, MD, MPH
Senior Director, Equity and Social Accountability

Lisa Howley, PhD, MEd
Senior Director, Strategic Initiatives and Partnerships
Series Lead

Sherese B. Johnson, MPH, PMP
Former Director, Public Health Initiatives
Director, Diversity, Equity, and Inclusion

Diana Lautenberger
Director, Gender Equity Initiatives

Ross McKinney, MD
Chief Scientific Officer
Executive Co-Sponsor

Norma Poll-Hunter, PhD
Senior Director, Workforce Diversity

Tiffani St.Cloud
Director, Educational Initiatives

Karey Sutton, PhD
Former Director of Research, AAMC Center for Health Justice
Former Director, Health Equity Research Work Force

Kamilah Weems, MS
Director, Strategic Initiatives and Partnerships
Series Co-Lead

Alison Whelan, MD
Chief Academic Officer
Executive Co-Sponsor

Titles and affiliations reflect those while people were active on the committee and may not be current.

Series Introduction

COMPETENCY-BASED EDUCATION

Competency-based education (CBE) is a developing approach to health professions education. The AAMC has a long history with CBE and defining the fundamentals for practicing in an increasingly complex health care system. Over the past 20 years, medical education has improved in many ways, including in how outcomes such as competencies are defined and used to guide teaching and learning. To support this kind of positive change, we offer the New and Emerging Areas in Medicine Series. The series frames competencies across the undergraduate, graduate, and continuing medical education continuum. This report includes an introduction to CBE and competencies in diversity, equity, and inclusion (DEI), including the historical context and importance of developing competence in this area and tactics for integrating this essential educational focus into the curriculum. Details about the development process and a glossary of terms are included as appendixes.

HISTORICAL CONTEXT OF DIVERSITY, EQUITY, AND INCLUSION COMPETENCIES

The goal of medical education is to prepare physicians to improve health and evolve as evidence evolves. Since the founding of the United States, there have been systemic health and health care inequities grounded in racism, sexism, homophobia, classism, and other forms of discrimination that still permeate our current health system. National data reports from the Agency for Healthcare Research and Quality and the Centers for Disease Control and Prevention show that racial and ethnic minority groups, people who live in poverty, rural and urban underserved communities, and LGBTQ communities disproportionately experience poor health and health care.[1] The current and the next generations of physicians need to be prepared to be responsive to the public health and societal needs of everyone.

Recent broad societal calls for social justice and the disparate impacts of the COVID-19 pandemic have added urgency to the need for improved integration of diversity, equity, inclusion, and anti-racism in medical education and training. Medical students and residents have also strongly expressed the need for curricular change. This change is particularly important in light of growing evidence that health care provider biases and behaviors can be significant factors in health care disparities.[2-9]

The origins of these inequities are often rooted in systemic racism and discrimination and are compounded by social risk factors that influence health (e.g., low-quality housing, food insecurity, poor access to transportation).[10-12] At the nexus of education and clinical care, academic medicine has a responsibility to address and mitigate the factors that drive racism and bias in health care and to prepare physicians who are culturally responsive and trained to address these issues.

While there has been significant progress in improving medical education in the past 20 years, medical schools and residency programs approach preparing students for culturally responsive care in variable and siloed ways. This content is often addressed in just one course or as a standalone elective. Some institutions struggle with finding faculty who can appropriately teach about culturally responsive care.

More than two decades ago, the Liaison Committee on Medical Education (LCME®) introduced an accreditation standard for medical schools supporting integrating cultural competence into the curriculum. The standard currently states that "faculty and students must demonstrate an understanding of the manner in which people of diverse cultures and belief systems perceive health and illness and respond to various symptoms, diseases, and treatments. Medical students should learn to recognize and appropriately address gender and cultural biases in health care delivery, while considering first the health of the patient."[13]

In 2012, the Accreditation Council for Graduate Medical Education (ACGME) also launched a Clinical Learning Environment Review (CLER) program as a part of its Next Accreditation System (NAS). This program includes health care disparities as one of its six focus areas. Also, within the NAS, individual specialties include a variety of milestones (outcomes) related to addressing social determinants of health, cultural humility, and advocating for health equity (acgme.org). More recently, the ACGME has established a new initiative, Equity Matters, which aims to "drive change within graduate medical education (GME) by increasing physician workforce diversity, and building safe and inclusive learning environments, while promoting health equity by addressing racial disparities in health care and overall population health."[14]

The Accreditation Council for Continuing Medical Education (ACCME) recently convened a task force to understand the scope of diversity, equity, and inclusion activities in the continuing education community and make recommendations for further action (accme.org). The member boards of the American Board of Medical Specialties (ABMS) are addressing DEI in various ways, from efforts related to governance to certifying examinations and continuing certification programs (abms.org).

In conjunction with the efforts by local programs and by accrediting and certification bodies, further work is needed to align DEI efforts across the continuum and, ultimately, develop physicians who are more fully equipped to address inequities in health care and who value diversity in all its forms. These competencies build on existing knowledge, acknowledge current efforts in academic medicine, and provide specific outcomes expected of students, residents, and faculty as they continue to grow and learn.

Cross-Continuum Competencies: Diversity, Equity, and Inclusion

ORGANIZATION OF THE COMPETENCIES

These competencies were developed over 24 months through an iterative process with extensive feedback from people engaged in health professions education, faculty development, research, direct patient care, and experts in DEI. (See Appendix A for details.) The competencies are organized into three domains — (1) Diversity, (2) Equity, and (3) Inclusion — and three tiers that represent developmental stages in physician development: (1) entry to residency or recent medical school graduate, (2) entry to independent practice or recent residency graduate, and (3) experienced faculty physician responsible for educating students or residents.

INTENDED USES

These cross-continuum competencies help educators design or adapt curricula and help educators and learners in their individual professional development and DEI journeys. The competencies can supplement existing competencies by providing more detail and depth and guide DEI curricular and professional development, formative performance assessments, and cross-continuum collaborations and, ultimately, improve health care services and outcomes. They are not intended to be used for high-stakes assessments or accreditation of schools, programs, or institutions. Examples of intended uses include:

- Engaging health care professionals in collaborative DEI discussions, including cross-continuum and cross-discipline colleagues.
- Conducting gap analyses of local curricula and training programs.
- Self-assessing and planning individual professional development.
- Developing curricular learning objectives.
- Developing assessment tools.
- Furthering research and scholarship in medical education and DEI.
- Guiding the strategic integration of DEI into the formal curricula and the clinical learning environment.

CAVEATS

These important caveats further clarify the design, intent, and use of the cross-continuum competencies:

- Although building competence in DEI is a journey and not a destination, this work aims to provide a standard set of expectations or outcomes along the developmental continuum. New demands and advances in health care require all health professionals, whether at the beginning or end of their careers, to be learners and acquire new and refresh existing competencies.
- These competencies recognize the important impact physicians have at the individual patient, health care team, health system, and community levels. And in all cases, the intent is to clarify the role of the physician and what they should know, do, and value in relation to their own practice, their team, and their health care system.
- Important terms and phrases are defined in the glossary (Appendix B).
- Competencies related to systems-level changes, advocacy, policy changes, and role modeling may be aspirational for some, depending on their local environment, education, and training. As we did with other sets of competencies, we strove to reach consensus in the balance we struck between what some subject matter experts may consider below expectation and others may consider aspirational. We will continue to listen to and learn from our diverse communities as we work on the next iteration.
- The first set of competencies in this series, Quality Improvement and Patient Safety (QIPS),[15] includes a domain titled "health equity in QIPS," and two relevant competencies from that set are included here. We will update the full set of QIPS competencies soon to better reflect the progress made not only in health equity, but in the overall domains of quality and safety.
- The third tier of competencies is designed for those who teach or supervise students or residents in a clinical learning environment, not all physicians.

FEEDBACK ON THE COMPETENCIES

This work is dynamic, and the competencies should be considered with that in mind. We plan to review and regularly update the competencies based on feedback from the community and new evidence and evolving language in these domains. Please contact DEICompetencies@aamc.org to share feedback, resources, suggestions, and exemplars for teaching and learning.

RESOURCES AND TOOLS

The AAMC has several freely available resources to support teaching and learning the competencies, and we welcome your contributions to these growing collections:

- *MedEdPORTAL, The Journal of Teaching and Learning Resources*, Anti-racism in Medicine Collection[16] and the Diversity, Inclusion, and Health Equity[17] Collection.
- The Clinical Teaching and Learning Experiences collection.[18]
- *Cultural Competence Education for Students in Medicine and Public Health: Report of an Expert Panel.*[13]

Diversity, Equity, and Inclusion Competencies

DOMAIN I: DIVERSITY

Diversity "refers to the identities we carry. There are many kinds of diversity, based on race, gender, sexual orientation, class, age, country of origin, education, religion, geography, physical or cognitive abilities, or other characteristics. Valuing diversity means recognizing differences between people, acknowledging that these differences are a valued asset, and striving for diverse representation as a critical step towards equity."[19]

Entering Residency (Recent Medical School Graduate) or New to DEI Journey	Entering Practice (Recent Residency Graduate) or Advancing Along DEI Journey *All prior competencies +*	Faculty Physician Teaching and Leading or Continuing DEI Journey *All prior competencies +*
Advancing Diversity and Integration in Practice Knowledge and practices demonstrating that one values and understands how aspects of an individual's overlapping identities create unique lived experiences that may influence health and health care outcomes		
1a. Demonstrates evidence of self-reflection and how one's personal identities, biases, and lived experiences may influence one's perspectives, clinical decision-making, and practice	1b. Mitigates the effects of personal bias in clinical decision-making and delivery of patient care	1c. Role models how the practice of self-reflection can help with identifying and mitigating effects of personal biases
2a. Demonstrates the value of diversity by incorporating dimensions of diversity into the patient's health assessment and treatment plan	2b. Gathers and applies patient-identified demographic data to develop a comprehensive patient health assessment and treatment plan	2c. Role models and teaches how to collect and apply patient-identified demographic data to develop a comprehensive patient health assessment and treatment plan
3a. Demonstrates knowledge of the intersectionality of a patient's multiple identities and how each identity may result in varied and multiple forms of oppression or privilege related to clinical decisions and practice	3b. Applies knowledge of intersectionality to inform clinical decisions and practice	3c. Role models how knowledge of intersectionality informs clinical decision-making and practice
Advocating for a Diverse Health Care Team and System Actions that promote social, economic, educational, and policy changes that advocate for achieving optimal learning, health, and well-being within the health care team and the system		
4a. Analyzes policies and practices that promote and ensure diversity of the health care team	4b. Advocates for policies and practices that promote, build, and sustain diversity of the health care team	4c. Role models and teaches how to advocate for policies and practices that promote, build, and sustain diversity of the health care team
5a. Identifies the system-level policies, procedures, and practices that may or may not promote diversity and inclusion in the health care system	5b. Adheres to system-level policies, procedures, and practices that promote diversity and inclusion in the health care system	5c. Leads, advocates for, and/or participates in the development, implementation, and review of policies, procedures, and practices that promote diversity and inclusion in the health care system

DOMAIN II: EQUITY

Equity "refers to fairness and justice and is distinguished from equality. While equality means providing the same to all, equity requires recognizing that we do not all start from the same place because power is unevenly distributed. The process is ongoing, requiring us to identify and overcome uneven distribution of power as well as intentional and unintentional barriers arising from bias or structural root causes."[19]

Entering Residency (Recent Medical School Graduate) or New to DEI Journey	Entering Practice (Recent Residency Graduate) or Advancing Along DEI Journey *All prior competencies +*	Faculty Physician Teaching and Leading or Continuing DEI Journey *All prior competencies +*
Mitigating Stigma and Implicit and Explicit Biases Practices that mitigate implicit and explicit attitudes or stereotypes in favor of or against one person or group compared with another; biases may influence attitudes and behaviors adversely, leading to discriminatory practices, especially when clinicians and educators are faced with external pressure or limited time		
1a. Articulates how one's own identities, power, and privileges (e.g., professional hierarchy, culture, class, gender) influence interactions with patients, families, communities, and members of the health care team	1b. Seeks and acts upon feedback about how one's own identities, power, and privileges influence patients, families, communities, and members of the health care team	1c. Role models and teaches how to engage in reflective practices related to individual identities, power, and privileges to improve interactions with patients, families, communities, and members of the health care team
2a. Demonstrates knowledge about the role of explicit and implicit bias in delivery of high-quality care[1,2]	2b. Identifies and mitigates explicit and implicit biases that occur in clinical decision-making[1,2]	2c. Role models effective strategies to mitigate explicit and implicit biases that may negatively affect clinical decision-making[1,2]
Eliminating Inequities in Health Care Practices that measurably reduce population-level differences in health outcomes, disease burden, and the distribution or allocation of resources between majority and marginalized groups based on race, ethnicity, sex, sexual orientation, gender identity, intellectual and developmental ability, socioeconomic status, the physical (built) environment, geographic location, and psychosocial-, behavioral-, and health care-related factors		
3a. Describes the value of working in an interprofessional team, including patients, to identify and address social risk factors influencing health (e.g., food security, housing, utilities, transportation)	3b. Works collaboratively with an interprofessional team, including patients, to screen and refer patients for appropriate resources to address social determinants of health	3c. Role models collaborative practices for working with an interprofessional team to address social determinants of health affecting patients and communities
4a. Identifies systems of power, privilege, and oppression and their impacts on health outcomes (e.g., White privilege, racism, sexism, heterosexism, ableism, religious oppression)	4b. Makes collaborative care decisions based on an understanding of how systems of power, privilege, and oppression influence health care policies and patient health outcomes	4c. Teaches how systems of power, privilege, and oppression inform policies and practices and how to engage with systems to disrupt oppressive practices

(continued)

(continued)

5a. Describes how stratification (e.g., by race, ethnicity, primary language, socioeconomic status, LGBTQ identification) of quality measures can allow identification of health care disparities[1]	5b. Explores stratified quality improvement (QI) data for their patient population and uses these data to identify health care disparities[1]	5c. Describes how monitoring stratified QI data can help assess the risk of unintended consequences (e.g., widening the disparity gap) and uses stratified QI data to guide and monitor QI interventions[1]
6a. Explains the role of the health care system in identifying and meeting the local needs of the community (e.g., the role of the community health needs assessment or the community health improvement plan)	6b. Collaborates with a diverse interprofessional team within their system and with community members to meet identified community health needs	6c. Leads, formulates, and/or participates in interprofessional partnerships designed to improve community health needs
Practicing Anti-racism and Critical Consciousness in Health Care Educational and clinical practices that seek to revise and correct local, state, and national policies; institutional practices; and cultural misrepresentations that enable and perpetuate racial bias and race-based health care inequities		
7a. Describes past and current examples of racism and oppression (internalized, interpersonal, institutional, and structural) and their impact on trust, health, and health care	7b. Engages with the health care team and patients to identify the impacts of racism and oppression and challenges these behaviors and practices in the local setting	7c. Role models anti-racism in medicine and teaching, including strategies grounded in critical understanding of unjust systems of oppression
8a. Articulates race as a social construct that is a cause of health and health care inequities, not a risk factor for disease	8b. Identifies and corrects misuse of clinical tools and practices that substantiate race-based medicine	8c. Supports and participates in system-level solutions to end racist practices in education and clinical delivery that substantiate race-based medicine
9a. Describes the impact of various systems of oppression on health and health care (e.g., colonization, White supremacy, acculturation, assimilation)	9b. Collaborates to identify and act on system-level strategies to reduce the effects of various systems of oppression on health and health care	9c. Teaches and examines system-level strategies to remedy the impact of systems of oppression on health and health care
Advocating for Equity in Health and Health Care Practices that influence decision-makers and other vested groups and individuals to support or implement system-level policies and practices that contribute to realizing health equity		
10a. Describes public policy that promotes social justice and addresses social determinants of health	10b. Promotes social justice and engages in efforts to eliminate health care disparities	10c. Leads or participates in organizational and public policy approaches to promote social justice, eliminate health care disparities, and address social determinants of health

(continued)

(continued)

11a. Identifies and, if appropriate, refers patients to relevant community resources that promote health equity and improve the health of local communities and populations	11b. Uses resources that support population health improvement strategies (e.g., systems and policy advocacy, program and policy development, other community-based interventions)	11c. Leads, participates in, or supports interprofessional partnerships with local health departments or community-based organizations to develop culturally responsive interventions

1. AAMC. *Quality Improvement and Patient Safety Competencies Across the Learning Continuum.* AAMC New and Emerging Areas in Medicine Series. Washington, DC: AAMC; 2019.
2. Glicksman E. Unconscious bias in academic medicine: overcoming the prejudices we don't know we have. *AAMCNews.* https://www.aamc.org/news-insights/unconscious-bias-academic-medicine-overcoming-prejudices-we-don-t-know-we-have. Published Sept. 27, 2016. Accessed April 26, 2022.

DOMAIN III: INCLUSION

Inclusion "refers to how our defining identities are accepted in the circles that we navigate. Belonging evolves from inclusion; it refers to the extent to which individuals feel they can be authentic selves and can fully participate in all aspects of their lives. Inclusion is a state of being valued, respected and supported. At the same time, inclusion is the process of creating a working culture and environment that recognizes, appreciates, and effectively utilizes the talents, skills and perspectives of every employee; uses employee skills to achieve the agency's objectives and mission; connects each employee to the organization; and encourages collaboration, flexibility and fairness. In total, inclusion is a set of behaviors (culture) that encourages employees to feel valued for their unique qualities and experience a sense of belonging."[19]

Entering Residency (Recent Medical School Graduate) or New to DEI Journey	Entering Practice (Recent Residency Graduate) or Advancing Along DEI Journey *All prior competencies +*	Faculty Physician Teaching and Leading or Continuing DEI Journey *All prior competencies +*
Fostering Belongingness Practices in the clinical and educational environments that result in individuals feeling valued for their authenticity and intersectionality. These practices create safe spaces where individuals can express themselves without a fear of retribution, feel validated for multiple identities, and feel valued for their unique contributions.		
1a. Identifies the practices and values that foster belongingness in partnership with a diverse health care team and patient population (e.g., authenticity, respect, support)	1b. Applies the norms, practices, and values that foster belongingness in partnership with a diverse health care team and patient population	1c. Role models and teaches norms, practices, and values that foster belongingness in partnership with a diverse health care team and patient population
2a. Demonstrates moral courage, self-advocacy, and allyship when facing and/or witnessing injustice (e.g., microaggression, discrimination, racism)	2b. Practices moral courage, self-advocacy, allyship, and being an active bystander or upstander to address injustices	2c. Role models moral courage, self-advocacy, allyship, and being an active bystander or upstander to address and prevent injustices

(continued)

(continued)

3a. Seeks mentorship or trusted peers for ongoing consultation and support of professional identity formation, professional development, and well-being	3b. Actively mentors and/or engages with trusted peers for continuous professional development, growth, and well-being	3c. Role models a growth mindset and how to leverage professional networks to enhance professional identity formation
Providing Culturally Responsive Patient Care Practices that promote inclusive and collaborative written and spoken communication that help patients, families, and health care teams understand and actively integrate health care information		
4a. Describes and demonstrates health literacy universal precautions aimed at supporting all patients' efforts to improve their health[1]	4b. Practices health literacy universal precautions in spoken and written communications with all patients and caregivers[1]	4c. Role models and teaches health literacy universal precautions[1]
5a. Uses language-interpretive services to ensure quality and safe patient care	5b. Demonstrates how to work collaboratively with language interpreters to ensure quality and safe patient care	5c. Role models and teaches when and how to integrate interpretive services into practice and teaches alternative strategies to ensure quality and safe patient care
6a. Practices cultural humility and, when appropriate, provides culturally relevant resources to patients	6b (and 6a). Practices cultural humility and, when appropriate, provides culturally relevant resources to patients	6c. Teaches or role models the importance of practicing cultural humility and providing appropriate culturally relevant resources to patients
Advocating for Inclusive Practices and a Healthy and Inclusive Physical (Built) Environment Practices that ensure patients, families, and communities have an equal voice and equal access to services and resources needed for optimal patient care		
7a. Differentiates between inclusive and exclusive policies and practices within the local health care system to ensure people from a variety of backgrounds and abilities have equal access to services and resources	7b. Upholds inclusive policies and practices and works to mitigate exclusionary ones (e.g., reports incidences and suggests improvements) so that people from a variety of backgrounds and abilities have equal access to services and resources	7c. Actively contributes to creating an environment that ensures people from a variety of backgrounds and abilities have equal access to services and resources
8a. Explains how structural aspects of the physical (built) environment can promote or inhibit inclusion	8b. Identifies opportunities to improve the physical (built) environment to foster a more inclusive health care environment	8c. Role models how to recognize and implement changes to the physical (built) environment to support a more inclusive health care environment

1. Brega AG, Barnard J, Mabachi NM, et al. *AHRQ Health Literacy Universal Precautions Toolkit, Second Edition*. Agency for Healthcare Research and Quality; 2015. AHRQ publication 15-0023-EF.

Curricular Models for Integrating and Improving Diversity, Equity, and Inclusion in Medical Education

Caring for Patients With Intellectual or Developmental Disabilities (IDD): The Introduction of the Standardized Patient With IDD

University of Tennessee Health Science Center College of Medicine Chattanooga
Rick Rader, MD, Director of the Habilitation Center, Orange Grove Center

Medical schools have traditionally used “standardized patients” (SPs), who are usually trained laypeople or actors hired to play the role of patients or actual patients hired to share their own lived experiences. A unique variation on that approach is to hire people with intellectual and developmental disabilities as SPs, and the Orange Grove Center has been doing just that since 1995. It includes four people diagnosed with Down syndrome, autism, Fragile X syndrome, or Williams syndrome in its SP program every year. Three of the SPs are verbal, and one uses an electronic communication device. All have been trained to report the onset of an array of symptoms to help guide medical students through the history-taking process and the physical examination, and they respond to questions posed by the medical students. The symptoms include pain in the lower-right abdomen, difficulty swallowing, recent onset of confusion, and spontaneous episodes of crying. In addition, the SPs encourage students to seek understanding about their lives, including their social dynamics, living arrangements, employment, stressors, and goals. The educational experience gives students the opportunity to learn how to communicate more effectively with and about this patient population, create a sensory-friendly environment, and include the assistance of a direct-support professional or caregiver, who is also present during the history taking and physical exam. Experiencing the challenges and rewards of successfully interacting with an individual with a complex disability increases medical students' self-confidence and appreciation of the role of implicit bias in health care. This educational activity aligns with many AAMC DEI Competencies, including Diversity 1-3, Equity 1-4, and Inclusion 1, 2, 4, 7, and 8.

Sexual and Gender Minority Health Faculty Development Modules

Harvard Medical School
John Dalrymple, MD, Alex Keuroghlian, MD, MPH, and Jennifer Potter, MD, Co-Directors of the Sexual and Gender Minority Health Equity Initiative

In 2018, Harvard Medical School launched a three-year Sexual and Gender Minority (SGM) Health Equity Initiative to integrate SGM health content across the curriculum. Early participant surveys demonstrated the need for a parallel curriculum to educate faculty in core SGM health content while simultaneously teaching them strategies for creating a curricular context in which all students can acquire requisite SGM health knowledge and skills. After establishing a set of faculty competencies encompassing both core SGM health content and how to create an affirming learning environment, the co-directors of the initiative created a series of nine online, interactive professional development modules for faculty. Many SGM health competencies addressed in these modules align closely with the AAMC DEI Competencies.

For example, Module 3: Implicit Bias and Power Imbalances aligns with Diversity Competencies 1, 2, 4, 7, and 9. It considers how unconscious bias and assumptions about SGM people may negatively affect health care outcomes for patients and educational outcomes for students, how physician-patient and faculty-student power imbalances may also negatively affect these outcomes, and how to mitigate potential adverse effects of implicit bias and power imbalances. Module 4: Sensitive and Affirming Communication addresses how to interact respectfully with all members of the health care team and patients regardless of gender identity, gender expression, sexual orientation, and sex development (Inclusion 1) and how to respond productively after a misstep (Inclusion 2). Module 6: How to Weave Intersectional Identities and Lived Experiences Into Cases and Case Presentations Without Stereotyping or Causing Offense reviews benefits and pitfalls of doing that weaving and describes how to responsibly include SGM identities and other characteristics (Diversity 1-3, Equity 2).

Faculty Development in Antiracist Pedagogy and Critical Consciousness

Icahn School of Medicine at Mount Sinai Center for Antiracism in Practice
Leona Hess, PhD, MSW, Founder and Co-Director; Jay Johnson, CHES, Education Program Manager; Joseph Truglio, MD, MPH, Director of Clinical Education; and Ann-Gel Palermo, DrPH, MPH, Co-Director

Through the Center for Antiracism in Practice (CAP) at the Icahn School of Medicine at Mount Sinai, a longitudinal "curriculum clinic" series was developed to build capacity for the ongoing practice of anti-racist pedagogy and critical consciousness within all courses and clerkships. The curriculum clinic journey aims to disrupt the perpetuation of racist ideologies and practices in all aspects of the curriculum, including teachers, learners, and content. The series consists of three interactive workshops, with pre- and post-session exercises, followed by ongoing one-on-one sessions with a CAP facilitator. Workshop 1 prepares participants to identify the manifestations of racism and White supremacy within their courses and explores how the biomedical model promotes a biological understanding of race (Equity 7 and 8; Inclusion 6). Workshop 2 guides participants in describing the impact of racism and White supremacy on learners and their future patients (Equity 9). In Workshop 3, participants identify concrete change targets within their courses and begin to develop alternative, anti-racist policies and practices. After completing the three workshops, participants work one-on-one with CAP facilitators to implement and assess the effectiveness of anti-racist pedagogy, policies, and practices within their courses. Throughout the series, participants use a course self-assessment tool, still under development, that is an inquiry-based guide with an anti-racist approach for assessing teaching and learning design practices and the impact of those practices. The tool promotes ongoing critical self-reflection and personal growth and provides strategies for course redesign and correction as they relate to the teacher, learner, and course content (Diversity 1).

Biomedical, Behavioral, Social Sciences, and Medical Ethics Curriculum

University of Texas Health Science Center at San Antonio Joe R. and Teresa Lozano Long School of Medicine
Chiquita A. Collins, PhD, MA, Chief Diversity Officer, Vice Dean for Inclusion and Diversity

There is growing recognition of the need to address the deleterious effects of systemic forms of bias on health — widely documented in the scientific literature — within medical education. At the Long School of Medicine, first-year medical students are introduced to an intensive and robust preclinical curriculum that includes a Medicine, Behavior and Society (MBS) module, which increases the fundamental understanding of social science issues related to medicine (e.g., ethics, humanism, professionalism). The module addresses relevant theories about and methods for increasing awareness and understanding of nonbiological factors that disproportionately contribute to adverse health outcomes, especially in underserved and marginalized populations (Equity 4, 5, 8, and 9).

Topics include the social construction of race, historical and contemporary forms of systemic discrimination, social determinants of health, patients' experiences, race-based medicine, power differentials, and advancing health equity. Case studies and various educational modalities are used to examine the intersectionality of race, gender, and socioeconomic status and other social identities (Diversity 3). For example, students participate in a poverty simulation where they are grouped into families of one to five people, assigned the role of a family member, and tasked with getting through a simulated month, separated into four 15-minute weeks during the on-day simulation session. Students are required to accomplish instrumental activities of daily living (IADLs), such as managing finances, transportation to work, and applying for public benefits and subsidies. Self-reflection, small- group dialogue, supplementary readings, and toolkits are also used as experiential learning tools (e.g., Women of Color Initiative, aamc.org/data-reports/women-of-color).

Appendix A. Development Process and Survey Questions

DEVELOPMENT PROCESS

There is no single standard approach to the development of competencies, but there are some preferred steps:

1. Define the scope of the competencies or the construct.
2. Engage diverse participants and collect data to understand the nature of the construct. How do high performers perform? How do those who achieve positive results behave in practice? Gather data through literature reviews, focus groups, and electronic surveys of subject matter experts.
3. Draft the competencies.
4. Have reactor panels of subject matter experts, patients, front-line clinicians, and educators review multiple drafts of competencies.
5. Importantly, review and update competencies periodically to keep pace with changes in clinical and educational practices.

In early 2020, the AAMC Diversity, Equity, and Inclusion Advisory Committee convened to begin drafting domains and competencies. The committee continued to meet virtually to develop a first draft. We took several approaches to collecting feedback.

We used a modified Delphi method to refine the competencies and increase participant input. This included developing a questionnaire of standard items (see the Survey Questions on page 18), conducting iterative email rounds with that questionnaire, collecting individual and group feedback between rounds, and summarizing the findings. An electronic questionnaire inviting feedback about the initial domains and competencies was initially distributed to 255 people from November 2020 through January 2021. Those who received that questionnaire included people engaged in health professions education, faculty development, research, direct patient care, and experts in DEI.

We used the feedback from the first iteration to revise the domains and the competencies and made multiple changes to the competencies across the three tiers and within all domains. The second questionnaire was sent in April 2021 to 301 people and included the same questions as the first version and a revised set of domains and competencies. The second questionnaire also asked respondents to indicate whether their primary educational focus is undergraduate medical education (UME), graduate medical education (GME), or continuing medical education/continuing professional development (CME/CPD).

The response rates for the first and second surveys were 73.3% and 57.1%, respectively. We analyzed the mixed-methods data from the two surveys and further revised the competencies.

We also held focus groups with a select group of medical school deans and medical educators directly involved in developing DEI curricula.

Overall, there was a more favorable response to the second questionnaire, with an average score across all Likert scale items 4% higher than the score for the first questionnaire, indicating, according to one medical educator respondent, the competencies "will be helpful to them as they educate students, residents and/or physician faculty." We then shared the final draft of the competencies again with the Advisory Committee for further refinement. The final version 1.0 of the AAMC DEI Competencies is on pages 7-12.

SURVEY QUESTIONS

Respondents, including focus group members and reactor panelists, reviewed the draft domains and related competencies and answered the following standard questions about each domain:

1. Tier: For use in curriculum development, does this set of draft competencies reflect observable abilities at the appropriate level for entering residency (recent medical school graduate), entering practice (recent residency graduate), or serving in a faculty or leadership role? Response Options: 1—No, not at all; 3—Somewhat; 5—Yes, definitely. Please describe your response. Explain how the competencies within this domain can be assessed. Are they observable?
2. Comprehensive: Does the set of draft competencies listed above reflect all specific knowledge, skills, values, and attitudes that are relevant to this domain? Response Options: 1—No, not at all; 3—Somewhat; 5—Yes, definitely. Please describe your response. Explain how these competencies are inclusive of all knowledge, skills, values, and attitudes within this domain.

3. Granularity: Does the language reflect an optimal level of granularity? Response Options: 1—No, not at all; 3—Somewhat; 5—Yes, definitely. Please describe your response. Can we be more specific in certain areas or add more detail? Are these competencies too granular?
4. Please provide general feedback on this subset of competencies.

At the end of the questionnaire, respondents were asked to consider the full set of draft competencies in the three DEI domains and answer the following questions:

1. Consider the entire set of competencies together. What, if anything, is missing? (open-ended)
2. How can we assist the medical education community with developing and supporting curricular and professional development activities that support these competencies in diversity, equity, and inclusion? (open-ended)

Appendix B.
Glossary of Select Terms

Many terms and definitions used throughout the DEI Competencies are listed below. The majority are taken from *Advancing Health Equity: A Guide to Language, Narrative and Concepts.*[19] That guide provides additional background and explanation for these terms, as well as for many others not listed here. Footnote callouts refer to citations in the references section that follows the glossary.

ableism: "Discrimination of people with disabilities based on the belief that typical abilities are superior. Like racism and sexism, ableism classifies entire groups of people as 'less than,' and structures opportunity to advantage some and disadvantage others."[19]

ally: "Someone who makes the commitment and effort to recognize their privilege (based on gender [identity], class, race, sexual [orientation], etc.) and work in solidarity with oppressed groups in the struggle for justice. Allies understand that it is in their own interest to end all forms of oppression, even those from which they may benefit in concrete ways."[19]

anti-racism: "The active process of naming and confronting racism by changing systems, organizational structures, policies and practices and attitudes, so that power is redistributed and shared equitably. ... Anti-racism is a strategy to achieve racial justice. An antiracist is someone who is supporting an antiracist policy through their actions or expressing antiracist ideas."[19]

assimilationist: "One who is expressing the racist idea that a racial group is culturally or behaviorally inferior and is supporting cultural or behavioral enrichment programs to develop that racial group with the goal that the group would then be better able to blend within the dominant group."[19]

class: "Relations of power among networked/organized social groups that direct society's major institutions (such as corporations and government authorities), material resources and investments. Classism is the systematic oppression of subordinated class groups, held in place by attitudes that rank people according to economic status, family lineage, job status, level of education and other divisions."[19]

colonization: "Some form of invasion, dispossession, and subjugation of a people. The invasion need not be military; it can begin — or continue — as geographical intrusion in the form of agricultural, urban, or industrial encroachments. The result of such incursion is the dispossession of vast amounts of lands from the original inhabitants. This is often legalized after the fact. The long-term result of such massive dispossession is institutionalized inequality. The colonizer/colonized relationship is by nature an unequal one that benefits the colonizer at the expense of the colonized."[20]

culture: "Set of shared attitudes, values, goals and practices that characterize an institution, organization or group. Culture is transmitted and reinforced through tradition, art, language and ritual, among other practices. It has also been defined more broadly as a social system of meaning and custom by a group of people to assure its adaptation and survival."[19]

disability: "Any condition of the body or mind (impairment) that makes it more difficult for the person with the condition to do certain activities (activity limitation) and interact with the world around them (participation restrictions)."[21]

discrimination: "Treatment of an individual or group based on their actual or perceived membership in a social category, usually used to describe unjust or prejudicial treatment on the grounds of race, age, sex, gender, ability, socioeconomic class, immigration status, national origin or religion. Discrimination by default positions some groups to have more advantages, opportunities, resources, protections than others based on a given social characteristic or combination of social characteristics that are differentially valued."[19]

diversity: "Refers to the identities we carry. There are many kinds of diversity, based on race, gender, sexual orientation, class, age, country of origin, education, religion, geography, physical or cognitive abilities, or other characteristics. Valuing diversity means recognizing differences between people, acknowledging that these differences are a valued asset, and striving for diverse representation as a critical step towards equity."[19]

equity: "Refers to fairness and justice and is distinguished from equality. While equality means providing the same to all, equity requires recognizing that we do not all start from the same place because power is unevenly distributed. The process is ongoing, requiring us to identify and overcome uneven distribution of power as well as intentional and unintentional barriers arising from bias or structural root causes."[19]

ethnicity: "Social construct and category based on shared geography, language, ancestry, traditions or history. The boundaries of authenticity (that is, who or what 'counts' in recognizing members of an ethnic group) are often changeable and dependent on generational, social, political and historical situations."[19]

experienced faculty physician: A person with an MD or DO degree who has completed residency and at least three years of independent practice and teaches or supervises learners, either paid or volunteer, full- or part-time.

explicit bias: "The traditional conceptualization of bias. With explicit bias, individuals are aware of their prejudices and attitudes toward certain groups. Positive or negative preferences for a particular group are conscious."[22]

gender: "The social, psychological, and emotional traits, attitudes, norms and behaviors, often influenced by society's expectations, that classify someone as man, woman, both, or neither."[19]

gender identity: "How people conceptualize themselves as gendered beings, including one's innate and personal experience of gender. This may or may not align with one's gender expression or biological sex."[19]

growth mindset: "Individuals who believe their talents can be developed (through hard work, good strategies, and input from others) have a growth mindset. They tend to achieve more than those with a more fixed mindset (those who believe their talents are innate gifts)."[23]

health care inequities: "A measurable, systemic, avoidable and unjust difference in health care access, utilization, quality and outcomes between groups, stemming from differences in levels of social advantage and disadvantage."[19]

health equity: "The absence of avoidable, unfair, or remediable differences among groups of people, whether those groups are defined socially, economically, demographically or geographically or by other means of stratification. 'Health equity' or 'equity in health' implies that ideally everyone should have a fair opportunity to attain their full health potential and that no one should be disadvantaged from achieving this potential."[19]

health literacy: "Used to describe the ability of individuals to locate, understand, interpret, and apply health information to guide their decisions and behavior."[19]

health literacy universal precautions: "Health literacy universal precautions are the steps that practices take when they assume that all patients may have difficulty comprehending health information and accessing health services."[24]

implicit bias: "Also known as unconscious bias, refers to attitudes or stereotypes that are outside our awareness but nonetheless affect our understanding, our interactions, and our decisions. Researchers have found that we all harbor automatic associations — both positive and negative — about other people based on characteristics such as race, ethnicity, gender, age, social class, and appearance. These unconscious associations may influence our feelings and attitudes and result in involuntary discriminatory practices, especially under demanding circumstances."[25]

inclusion: "Refers to how our defining identities are accepted in the circles that we navigate. Belonging evolves from inclusion; it refers to the extent to which individuals feel they can be authentic selves and can fully participate in all aspects of their lives. Inclusion is a state of being valued, respected and supported. At the same time, inclusion is the process of creating a working culture and environment that recognizes, appreciates, and effectively utilizes the talents, skills and perspectives of every employee; uses employee skills to achieve the agency's objectives and mission; connects each employee to the organization; and encourages collaboration, flexibility and fairness. In total, inclusion is a set of behaviors (culture) that encourages employees to feel valued for their unique qualities and experience a sense of belonging."[19]

intersectionality: "Leading feminist and social justice theories and practices acknowledge that intersectionality, first coined by Kimberlé Crenshaw, as legal terminology to recognize the unique experiences and legal challenges of Black women, whom as a group experienced both racism and sexism. It is the ongoing examination of the overlapping systems of oppression and discrimination that communities face based on race, gender, ethnicity, ability, etc. It is our role to continuously examine the multiple forms and kinds of intersectional exclusions. The call for an anti-racist health care system — one which recognizes and addresses the intersectionality of systems of oppression — amplifies every day."[19]

LGBTQ: "An acronym for 'lesbian, gay, bisexual, transgender and queer.'"[26]

marginalized: "Process experienced by those under- or unemployed or in poverty, unable to participate economically or socially in society, including the labor market, who thereby suffer material as well as social deprivation."[19]

microaggression: "Everyday verbal, nonverbal and environmental slights, snubs or insults, whether intentional or unintentional, which communicate hostile, derogatory or negative messages to persons targeted solely for their membership in historically marginalized groups."[19]

oppression: "Unjust or cruel exercise of power or authority; the product of injustice. But also, as Iris Marion Young explains, '... the vast and deep injustices some groups suffer as a consequence of often unconscious assumptions and reactions of well-meaning people in ordinary interactions, media, and cultural stereotypes, and structural features of bureaucratic hierarchies and market mechanisms — in short the normal processes of everyday life.'"[19]

privilege: "A set of advantages systemically conferred on a particular person or group of people."[19]

race: "System of categorizing people that arises to differentiate groups of people in hierarchies to advantage some and disadvantage others. Stated another way, race is a social construct or [, according to M. Desmond and M. Emirbayer,] 'a symbolic category [actively created and recreated, rather than pre-given], based on phenotype or ancestry and constructed to specific racial and historical contexts, that is misrecognized as a natural category.' While often assumed to be a biological classification, based on physical and genetic variation, racial categories do not have a scientific basis."[19]

racism: "As defined by Camara Jones, 'Racism is a system of structuring opportunity and assigning value based on phenotype ('race'), that unfairly disadvantages some individuals and communities, unfairly advantages other individuals and communities, and undermines realization of the full potential of the whole society through the waste of human resources.' Racism can operate at different levels: structural, institutional, interpersonal and internalized."[19]

- **structural racism:** "Refers to the totality of ways in which societies foster racial discrimination through mutually reinforcing systems of housing, education, employment, earnings, benefits, credit, media, health care, and criminal justice. These patterns and practices in turn reinforce discriminatory beliefs, values, and distribution of resources," as defined by Zinzi Bailey et al.[19]
- **institutional racism:** "Discriminatory treatment, unfair policies and practices, and inequitable opportunities and impacts within organizations and institutions, based on race. Individuals within institutions take on the power of the institution when they act in ways that advantage and disadvantage people, based on race." [19]
- **interpersonal racism:** "The expression of racism between individuals. These are interactions occurring between individuals that often take place in the form of harassing, racial slurs or racial jokes. It may also take more subtle forms of unequal treatment, including micro-aggressions."[19]
- **internalized racism:** "Acceptance by members of stigmatized races of negative messages about their own abilities and intrinsic worth."[19]

role model: "One who serves as an example for others by demonstrating the behavior associated with a particular social position or profession."[20]

sexism: "Discrimination based on sex, typically the belief that cisgender males are inherently superior to all other genders."[19]

sexual orientation: "An inherent or immutable enduring emotional, romantic or sexual attraction to other people. Note: an individual's sexual orientation is independent of their gender identity."[19]

social determinants of health: "Refer to the underlying community-wide social, economic and physical conditions in which people are born, grow, live, work and age. They affect a wide range of health, functioning, and quality-of-life outcomes and risks. These determinants and their unequal distribution according to social position, result in differences in health status between population groups that are avoidable and unfair."[19]

stereotype: "Assignment of assumed characteristics or attributes to the members of a given group (e.g., by ethnicity, nationality, class, or other status/identities). It occurs in a variety of historical representations or expressions that can cause trauma and racial injury by 'othering' groups and denying people their individuality, culture and humanity."[19]

stigma: "Elements of labeling, stereotyping, separating, status loss and discrimination co-occurring in a power situation that allows these processes to unfold."[19]

systems of oppression: "The combination of prejudice and institutional power which creates a system that discriminates against some groups (often called 'target groups') and benefits other groups (often called 'dominant groups')."[19]

upstander: "A person who speaks or acts in support of an individual or cause, particularly someone who intervenes on behalf of a person being attacked or bullied."[27]

White supremacy: "Historically based, institutionally perpetuated system of exploitation and oppression of continents, nations, and people of color by White people and nations of European descent for the purpose of maintaining and defending a system of wealth, power and privilege."[19]

References

1. Agency for Healthcare Research and Quality. *2021 National Healthcare Quality and Disparities Report*. Rockville, MD: AHRQ. https://www.ahrq.gov/research/findings/final-reports/iomracereport/index.html. Accessed July 6, 2022.

2. Cooper LA, Roter DL, Carson KA, et al. The associations of clinicians' implicit attitudes about race with medical visit communication and patient ratings of interpersonal care. *Am J Public Health*. 2012;102(5):979-987. doi:10.2105/ajph.2011.300558.

3. Forgiarini M, Gallucci M, Maravita A. Racism and the empathy for pain on our skin. *Front Psychol* 2011;2:108. doi:10.3389/fpsyg.2011.00108.

4. Mossey JM. Defining racial and ethnic disparities in pain management. *Clin Orthop Relat Res*. 2011;469(7):1859-1870. doi:10.1007/s11999-011-1770-9.

5. Hall WJ, Chapman MV, Lee KM, et al. Implicit racial/ethnic bias among health care professionals and its influence on health care outcomes: a systematic review. *Am J Public Health*. 2015;105(12):e60-76. doi:10.2105/AJPH.2015.302903.

6. Schuster MA, Collins R, Cunningham WE. Perceived discrimination in clinical care in a nationally representative sample of HIV-infected adults receiving health care. *J Gen Intern Med*. 2005;20(9):807-813. doi:10.1111/j.1525-1497.2005.05049.x.

7. Sabin JA, Greenwald AG. The influence of implicit bias on treatment recommendations for 4 common pediatric conditions: pain, urinary tract infection, attention deficit hyperactivity disorder, and asthma. *Am J Public Health*. 2012;102(5):988-995. doi:10.2105/AJPH.2011.300621.

8. Schulman KA, Berlin JA, Harless W, et al. The effect of race and sex on physicians' recommendations for cardiac catheterization. *N Engl J Med*. 1999;340:618-626. doi:10.1056/NEJM199902253400806.

9. Centola D, Guilbeault D, Sarkar U, et al. The reduction of race and gender bias in clinical treatment recommendations using clinician peer networks in an experimental setting. *Nat Commun*. 2021;12:6585. doi:10.1038/s41467-021-26905-5.

10. Wallace M, Crear-Perry J, Richardson L, et al. Separate and unequal: structural racism and infant mortality in the US. *Health Place*. 2017;45:140-144. doi:10.1016/j.healthplace.

11. Dickinson KL, Roberts JD, Banacos N, et al. Structural racism and the COVID-19 experience in the United States. *Health Secur*. 2021;19(S1):S-14. doi:10.1089/hs.2021.0031.

12. Gachupin FC, Lee BR, Chipollini J, et al. Renal cell carcinoma surgical treatment disparities in American Indian/Alaska Natives and Hispanic Americans in Arizona. *Int J Environ Res Public Health*. 2022;19(3):1185. doi:10.3390/ijerph19031185.

13. AAMC, Association of Schools of Public Health. Expert Panel on Cultural Competence Education for Students in Medicine and Public Health. *Cultural Competence Education for Students in Medicine and Public Health: Report of an Expert Panel*. Washington, DC: AAMC and ASPH; 2012.

14. Accreditation Council for Graduate Medical Education. *ACGME Equity Matters*. Chicago, IL: AGCME. https://www.acgme.org/what-we-do/diversity-equity-and-inclusion/ACGME-Equity-Matters/. Accessed Feb. 24, 2022.

15. AAMC. *Quality Improvement and Patient Safety Competencies Across the Learning Continuum*. AAMC New and Emerging Areas in Medicine Series. Washington, DC: AAMC; 2019.

16. AAMC. Anti-racism in Medicine Collection. *MedEdPORTAL*. https://www.mededportal.org/anti-racism. Accessed Nov. 5, 2021.

17. AAMC. Diversity, Inclusion, and Health Equity Collection. *MedEdPORTAL*. https://www.mededportal.org/diversity-inclusion-and-health-equity. Accessed Nov. 5, 2021.

18. AAMC. Clinical Teaching and Learning Experiences. https://www.aamc.org/resource-library/clinical-teaching-and-learning-experiences. Accessed Nov. 5, 2021.

19. American Medical Association, AAMC. *Advancing Health Equity: A Guide to Language, Narrative and Concepts.* Washington, DC: American Medical Association; 2021. Accessed Nov. 21, 2021. https://www.ama-assn.org/system/files/ama-aamc-equity-guide.pdf

20. Racial Equity Tools. Racial equity tools glossary. https://www.racialequitytools.org/glossary. Accessed Nov. 21, 2021.

21. Centers for Disease Control and Prevention. Disability and health overview. https://www.cdc.gov/ncbddd/disabilityandhealth/disability.html. Accessed Nov. 21, 2021.

22. U.S. Department of Justice. *Understanding Bias: A Resource Guide.* Washington, DC: U.S. Department of Justice; 2015. https://www.justice.gov/crs/file/836431/download. Accessed Nov. 21, 2021.

23. Dweck CS. *Mindset: The New Psychology of Success.* New York: Random House; 2006.

24. Agency for Healthcare Research and Quality. *AHRQ Health Literacy Universal Precautions Toolkit.* Rockville, MD: AHRQ; April 2010. Updated September 2020. https://www.ahrq.gov/health-literacy/improve/precautions/index.html. Accessed Nov. 21, 2021.

25. AAMC, Kirwan Institute for the Study of Race and Ethnicity at The Ohio State University. *Proceedings of the Diversity and Inclusion Innovation Forum: Unconscious Bias in Academic Medicine — How the Prejudices We Don't Know We Have Affect Medical Education, Medical Careers, and Patient Health.* Washington, DC: AAMC; 2017. https://store.aamc.org/downloadable/download/sample/sample_id/168/.

26. Human Rights Campaign. Glossary of terms. https://www.hrc.org/resources/glossary-of-terms. Accessed Nov. 21, 2021.

27. Facing History and Ourselves. https://www.facinghistory.org/upstander. Accessed April 18, 2022.